Healthy, Heart-Smart Diet Recipes

A Helpful Cookbook of Low-calorie /
Low-carb Dish Ideas!

Table of Contents

Introduction

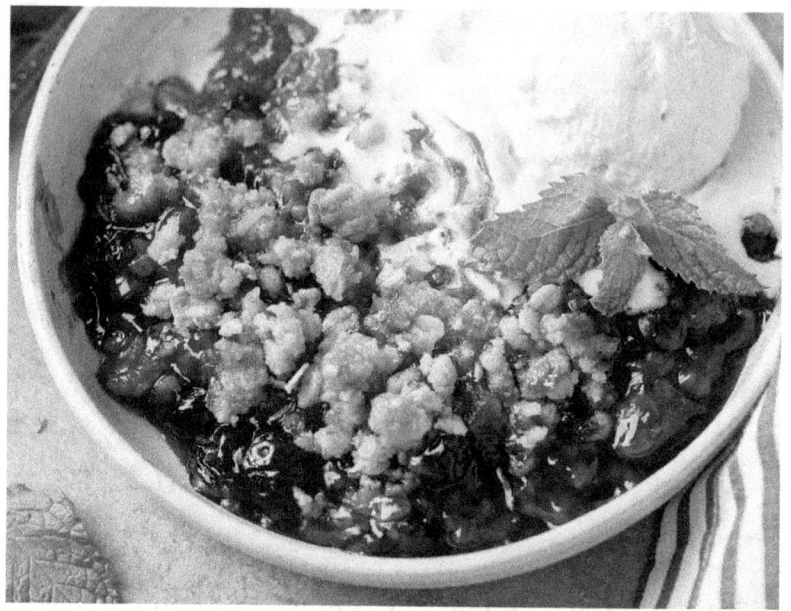

How will you make changes to support your diet, and still enjoy tasty foods? It can be done, and this cookbook will show you how.

Packaging single servings is helpful in dieting, especially if some in your household aren't on a diet. Prepare snacks, lunches, etc., ahead of time and repackage snacks so that you won't have the temptation of eating more of any snack or other food that could sabotage your diet.

Your family probably has tons of activities after school or play dates if they're younger. That makes it harder to plan meals. However, if you plan a week in advance, you can know just what is needed each evening. Ask your spouse and children, if you have them, what some of their favorite healthy foods are, so those can be included, too.

The more you cook at home, the more weight you will likely use. You'll be taking in fewer carbs and less sugar, because you'll know exactly how much is in every meal. Pre-packaged and restaurant meals are usually heavier in calories and are less nutritious, too.

You can even eat the same types of foods you eat out, but you're cooking them at home. You cook healthier than most restaurants do, so you'll be taking in less fat and more healthy foods.

When you begin shopping for and preparing healthy meals for weight loss, the pounds will more likely STAY off. Cooking diet-friendly meals will help your whole family to eat in a way that will keep everyone healthier and happier. Turn the page and let's get started!

1 – Mexi Breakfast Peppers

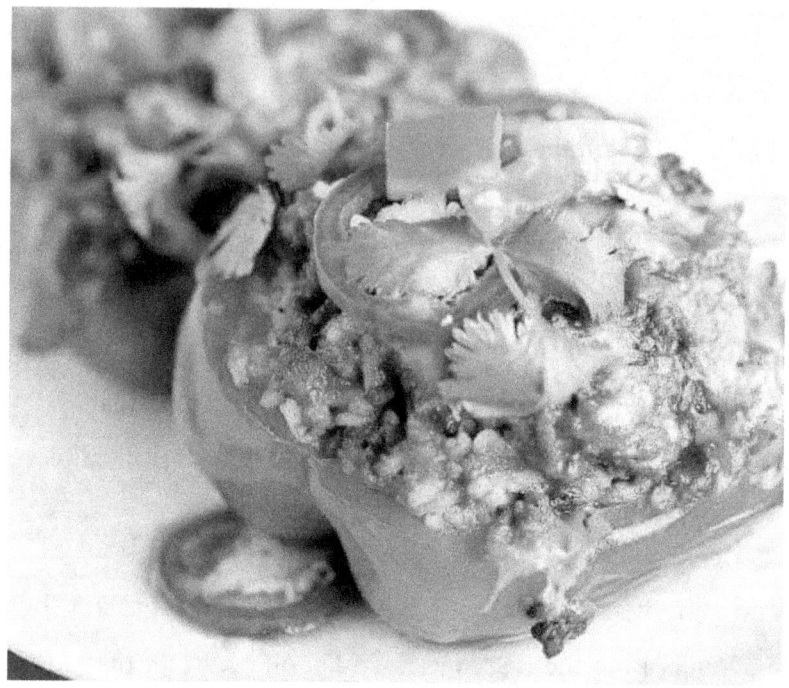

This healthy version of stuffed peppers uses red peppers, chorizo, ground beef and onions. When you fill the peppers with this delightful stuffing mixture, they look almost as good as they taste.

Makes 4 Servings

Cooking + Prep Time: 1/2 hour

Ingredients:

- 4 ounces of chorizo, beef and pork
- 4 oz. of beef, ground
- 1/2 cup of onions, chopped
- 1/4 cup of cheddar cheese shreds
- 3 whole eggs, large
- 2 sweet red peppers, medium

Instructions:

1. Preheat the oven to 400F. Line cookie sheet with aluminum foil.

2. Cook the chorizo. Stir it so you're breaking up the lumps, until it has browned, then drain off any excess fat.

3. Place ground beef and browned chorizo in large bowl. Combine with eggs, onion and cheese.

4. Cut the peppers lengthways in halves. Scoop out the seeds. Cut away the ribs.

5. Fill pepper halves with 1/4 meat mixture each. Place on cookie sheet. Bake for 25 to 30 minutes at 400F. Serve hot.

Nutrition Information

Amount Per Serving

Calories: 276.2

Total Fat: 17.3 g

Cholesterol: 53.2 mg

Sodium: 568.5 mg

Total Carbs: 13.5 g

Dietary Fiber: 3.4 g

Protein: 18.1 g

2 – Citrus Salad with Mint & Honey

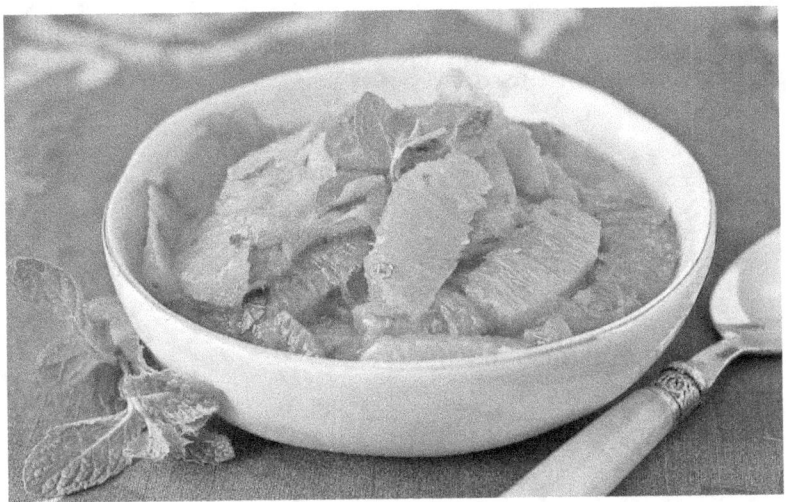

You can start the day off right with this bright, tasty dish that will wake up your senses. It's easy to make and the taste is unique and delectable, with its yummy honey dressing.

Makes 2 Servings

Cooking + Prep Time: 15 minutes

Ingredients:

- 1 navel orange
- 1 grapefruit
- 2 tsp. of honey, pure
- 4 fresh mint sprigs, small

Instructions:

1. Cut away peel and white-colored pith from orange and grapefruit. Slice fruits into circles.

2. Arrange slices on small, individual plates.

3. Use honey to drizzle and top with mint sprigs. Serve.

Nutrition Information

Amount Per Serving

Calories: 111.1

Total Fat: 5.0 g

Cholesterol: 0.0 mg

Sodium: 5.1 mg

Total Carbs: 16.8 g

Dietary Fiber: 2.7 g

Protein: 1.8 g

3 – Chorizo Breakfast Wrap

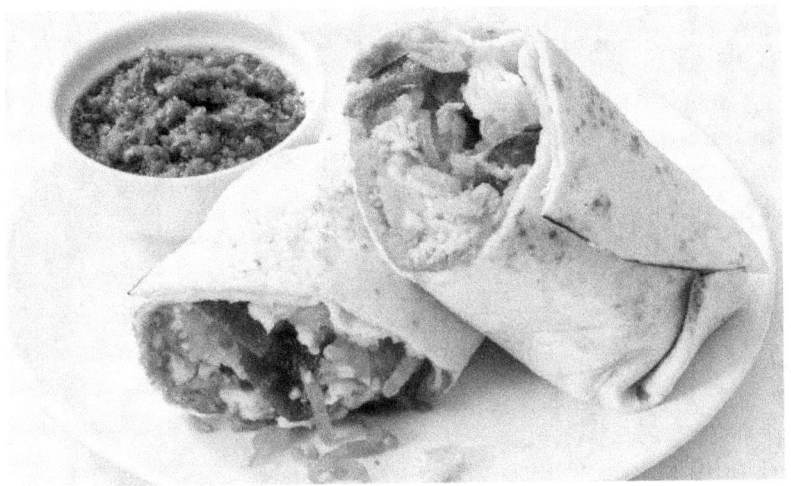

This is a great breakfast wrap that packs the flavor but not the calories, with its eggs, chorizo and mushrooms. It **Makes** getting up in the morning seem WORTH it.

Makes 2 Servings

Cooking + Prep Time: 15 minutes

Ingredients:

- 2 fresh eggs, raw, large
- 2 tbsp. of taco sauce, your favorite brand
- 2 oz. of beef and pork chorizo
- 1 serving of part-skim Queso Fresco

- 2 small tortillas, soft tacos, low carb
- 1/4 cup of egg substitute
- 1/4 cup of mushrooms, fresh

Instructions:

1. Cook mushrooms and chorizo together. Add the eggs and cheese.

2. Lightly toast the tortillas. Fill. Add salsa. Serve.

Nutrition Information

Amount Per Serving

Calories: 356.5

Total Fat: 20.7 g

Cholesterol: 218.4 mg

Sodium: 1,021.8 mg

Total Carbs: 13.8 g

Dietary Fiber: 6.1 g

Protein: 27.3 g

4 – Keto Breakfast Muffins

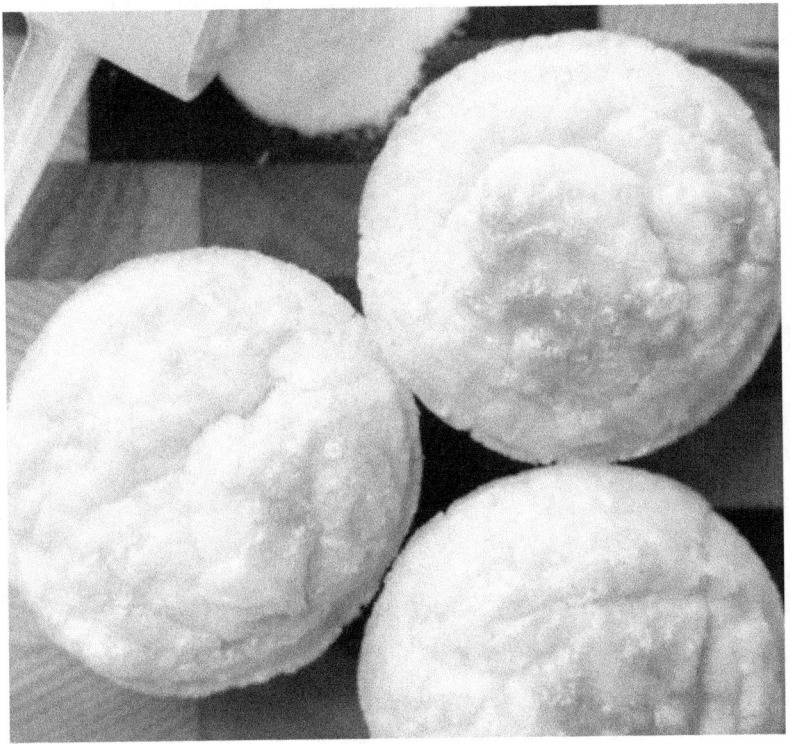

These are low carb muffins that still manage to be filling and fluffy. You can make them in sweet tastes or savory. In addition, you can change up some of the ingredients with your own healthy favorites.

Makes 1 Serving

Cooking + Prep Time: 5 minutes or less

Ingredients:

- Butter, unsalted
- 2 tsp. of coconut flour
- 1 egg, large
- 1 pinch of salt, kosher
- 1 pinch of baking soda
- 1 tsp. of sweetener, natural
- 1 tsp. of cinnamon, ground
- To top: butter, extra cinnamon and sweetener

Instructions:

1. Grease one ramekin with butter or coconut oil.

2. Mix all ingredients using a fork. Make sure it doesn't have any lumps.

3. Cook in microwave on the HIGH setting for 45 to 60 seconds. (You can also bake in 400F oven for 10-12 minutes, if you prefer.) Slice in half. Serve.

Nutrition Information

Amount Per Serving (1 keto muffin)

Calories 113 Calories from Fat 54

% Daily Value

Total Fat 6g 9%

Saturated Fat 2g 10%

Cholesterol 186mg 62%

Sodium 91mg 4%

Potassium 69mg 2%

Total Carbohydrates 5g 2%

Dietary Fiber 3g 12%

Protein 7g 14%

5 – Goat Cheese Omelet

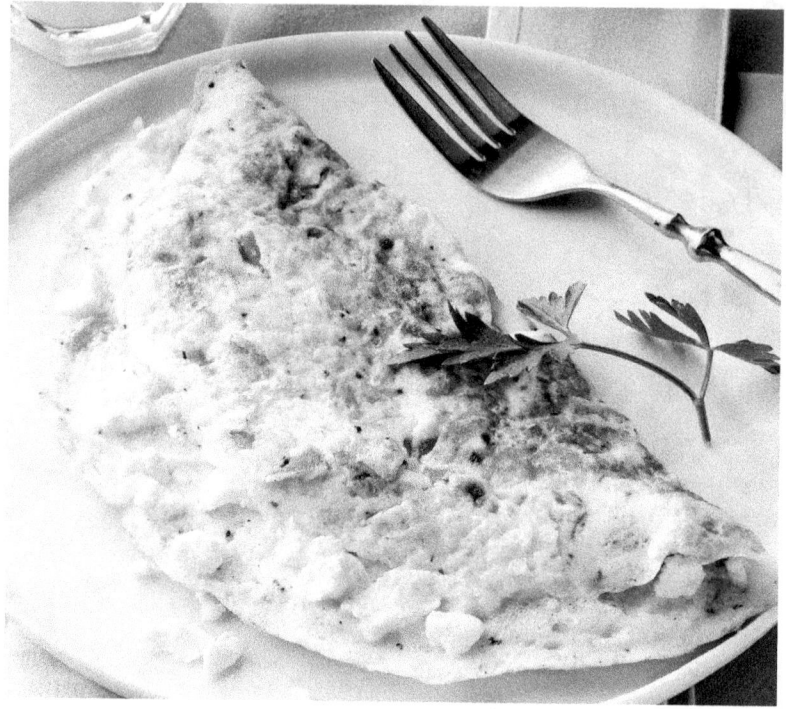

This is a simple and delicious omelet made from goat cheese, scallions and Dijon mustard, with lots of other healthy ingredients, too. The goat cheese gives the omelet a bit of a tart flavor that **Makes** it different from many others.

Makes 4 Servings

Cooking + Prep Time: 20 minutes

Ingredients:

- 8 eggs, large
- Salt, kosher, as desired
- Pepper, black, as desired
- 1 tbsp. of butter, unsalted
- 4 oz. of crumbled goat cheese, fresh
- 4 sliced scallions
- 3 tbsp. of oil, olive
- 1 tbsp. of vinegar, white wine
- 1 tsp. of mustard, Dijon
- 6 cups of arugula, baby
- 1 warmed baguette, small

Instructions:

1. Whisk 2 tbsp. of filtered water, eggs, 1/2 tsp. of kosher salt and 1/4 tsp. of black pepper together in a medium bowl.

2. Melt butter in non-stick skillet on med. heat. Cook eggs and do not stir them, till they start setting. This usually takes only two or three minutes.

3. Use a spatula to lift omelet edges. Tilt pan so uncooked egg flows to pan edges. Cook for about a minute, till eggs have set.

4. Sprinkle scallions and cheese on eggs. Fold 1/3 of omelet over center. Then fold the other 1/3 over. Cut into four pieces while still in pan.

5. Whisk vinegar, oil, mustard, 1/4 tsp of kosher salt and 1/4 tsp. of black pepper together. Drizzle this mixture over arugula. Serve with bread and omelet.

Nutrition Information

Serving Size: 1 serving

Amount Per Serving

Calories 126.4

Total Fat 8.4 g

Saturated Fat 3.5 g

Polyunsaturated Fat 0.7 g

Monounsaturated Fat 2.4 g

Cholesterol 192.0 mg

Sodium 120.4 mg

Potassium 53.2 mg

Total Carbohydrate 1.5 g

Dietary Fiber 0.0 g

Sugars 0.3 g

Protein 10.5 g

Here are some tasty, healthy recipes for lunch, dinner and side dishes...

6 – Stuffed Acorn Squash

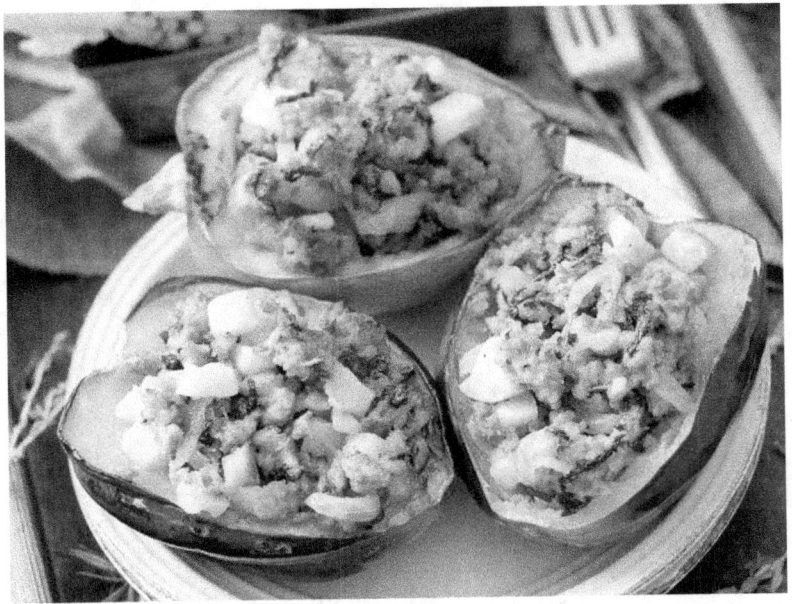

Sometimes it seems difficult to find healthy recipes that everyone in the family will enjoy. This squash is a meal my family loves, and the ingredients offer something for everyone.

Makes 8 Servings

Cooking + Prep Time: 1 & 1/2 hours

Ingredients:

- 4 acorn squash, medium
- 1 cup of halved tomatoes, cherry
- 1 lb. of Italian turkey sausage with removed link casings
- 1/2 lb. of sliced mushrooms, fresh
- 1 peeled, chopped apple, medium
- 1 chopped onion, small
- 2 tsp. of caraway seeds
- 2 tsp. of fennel seed
- 1/2 tsp. of sage leaves, dried
- 3 cups of baby spinach, fresh
- 1 tbsp. of minced thyme, fresh
- 1/4 tsp. of salt, kosher
- 1/8 tsp. of pepper, ground
- 8 oz. of chopped mozzarella cheese, fresh
- 1 tbsp. of vinegar, red wine

Instructions:

1. Preheat the oven to 400F. Cut the squash lengthways in halves. Remove the seeds and discard them.

2. Use a sharp knife to cut thin slices from bottoms of halves so they will lie flat. Place the squash in roasting pan with the hollow side facing down. Add 1/4 inch of hot water and the halved tomatoes. Leave uncovered and bake for 45 minutes.

3. Cook the sausage, dried seasonings, onion, apple and mushrooms on med. heat in skillet for 8 to 10 minutes till the sausage isn't pink any more. Break up sausage in crumbles and drain.

4. Add the spinach, kosher salt, ground pepper and thyme. Stir while cooking for two minutes. Then remove pan from heat.

5. Remove squash from the roasting pan. Drain the cooking liquid and reserve the tomatoes. Return the squash to the pan with the hollow side facing up.

6. Stir the reserved tomatoes, cheese and vinegar into the sausage mixture. Spoon this into the cavities in the squash. Bake for five to 10 minutes more till mixture has heated completely through and is pierced easily using a fork. Serve.

Nutrition Information

1 stuffed squash half: 302 calories

43mg cholesterol

10g fat (5g saturated fat)

42g carbohydrate

370mg sodium

7g fiber

11g sugars

15g protein

7 – Pork & Red Peppers

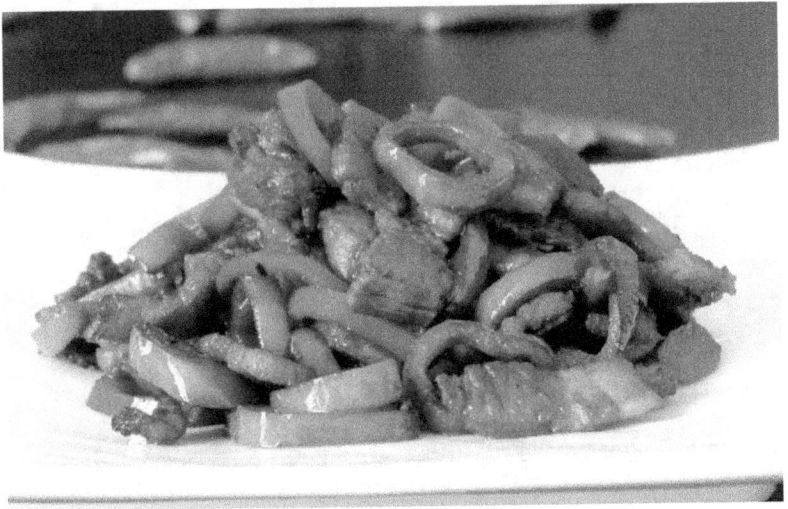

This is a great flavor combination, and low in calories and carbs! It offers pork, accented by sweet red peppers and garlic. The lemons give it a bright, fresh taste.

Makes 8 Servings

Cooking + Prep Time: 45 minutes + 3-4 hours marinating time

Ingredients:

- 4 peeled garlic cloves, large
- 1 & 1/2 tsp. of salt, coarse

- 2 tbsp. of oil, olive

- 1 tbsp. of black peppercorns, whole

- 2 lbs. of pork tenderloin, sliced in 1" medallions

- 2 julienned bell peppers, red

- 1 cup of wine, white

- 2 lemons, fresh

Instructions:

1. Mash 1 tbsp. of oil plus salt, peppercorns and garlic into fine-textured paste. Transfer it to large sized bowl.

2. Flatten pork medallions down to 1/4" thickness. Place in bowl with garlic mixture and toss to coat. Cover. Marinate for three to four hours in refrigerator.

3. Heat the rest of the oil in large-sized skillet on high heat. Add and stir pork and the rest of the garlic mixture. Brown the pork quickly, for about one minute per side. Remove the pan from heat. Set it aside.

4. Place the red peppers in skillet. Sauté for two to five minutes, till firm but tender. Pour the wine into skillet. Use it to scrape up any browned bits.

5. Reduce the heat down to low. Return the pork to the skillet. Cook for 10-15 more minutes, till internal temperature is 180F.

6. Slice 1 & 1/2 fresh lemons into circles. Transfer pepper and pork mixture to platter. Squeeze the juice from the last 1/2 fresh lemon over peppers and pork. Use lemon rounds to garnish. Serve.

Nutrition Information

Per Serving: 211 calories

7.6 g fat

6.7 g carbohydrates

24.3 g protein

74 mg cholesterol

423 mg sodium

8 – Chicken Taco Pie

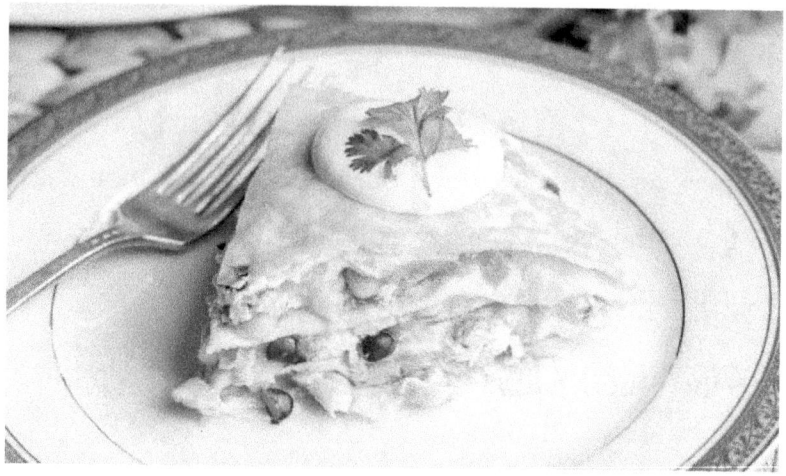

This recipe is one of my favorites to make, since I can do the putting together in the early morning and then pop it into my oven when everyone is home to eat dinner.

Makes 6 Servings

Cooking + Prep Time: 55 minutes

Ingredients:

- 1 x 8-oz. tube of crescent rolls, refrigerated
- 1 lb. of chicken, ground
- 1 packet of taco seasoning mixture
- 1 x 4-oz. can of green chilies, chopped

- 1/2 cup of water, filtered
- 1/2 cup of salsa, mild or hot, your choice
- 1/2 cup of Mexican cheese blend shreds
- 1 cup of lettuce, shredded
- 1 chopped small pepper, red, sweet
- 1 chopped small pepper, green
- 1 de-seeded, chopped tomato, medium
- 1 sliced green onion
- 2 tbsp. of jalapeno slices, pickled
- To serve: extra salsa and sour cream

Instructions:

1. Preheat the oven to 350F. Unroll the crescent dough. Separate it into triangles and press on to the bottom of pre-greased 9" pie pan, forming a crust. Seal the seams well. Bake till the crust is a golden-brown color. This usually takes about 15-20 minutes.

2. Cook the chicken on med. heat in large sized skillet till it isn't pink anymore. Break it into crumbles as you cook. Drain when lightly browned and in crumbles.

3. Add water, salsa, green chilies and taco seasoning. Bring to boil.

4. Spoon the mixture into your crust and sprinkle it with cheese. Bake till cheese melts, or about eight to 10 minutes.

5. Then top the pie with lettuce, red and green peppers, jalapenos and green onions. Garnish with extra salsa and sour cream and serve.

Nutrition Information

1 piece (calculated without the sour cream and the additional salsa):

17g fat (6g saturated fat)

328 calories

1122mg sodium

58mg cholesterol

5g sugars

25g carbohydrate

17g protein

1g fiber

9 – Cheese Broccoli Bake

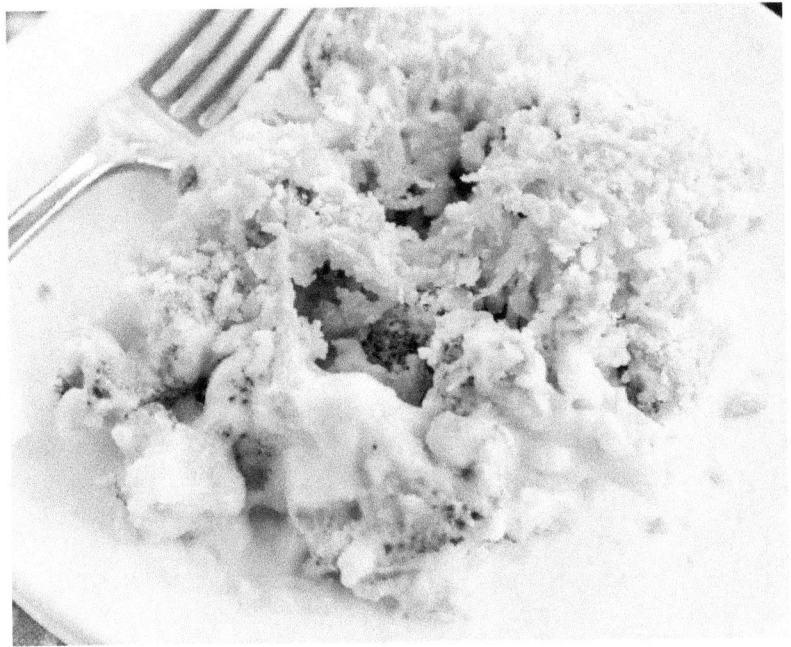

Do you or someone in your family love "bakes" but not the breadcrumbs? This is a different style of casserole, and you can leave out the eggs if you like. You can make many little alterations to this recipe, to make it a favorite for everyone.

Makes 7 Servings

Cooking + Prep Time: 50 minutes

Ingredients:

- 8 cups of broccoli, fresh
- 1/2 cup of butter, unsalted
- 2 tbsp. of flour, all-purpose
- 1 chopped onion, small
- 1 & 1/4 cups of milk, 2%
- Salt, kosher, as desired
- Pepper, ground, as desired
- 4 cups of Swiss cheese shreds
- 2 beaten eggs, large

Instructions:

1. Preheat the oven to 325F.

2. Place the broccoli in steamer over an inch of boiling, filtered water. Cover. Cook till firm but tender. Drain.

3. Melt the butter in sauce pan on med. heat. Add the flour and cook till it is bubbly.

4. Add and stir onion. Add milk gradually, while stirring thoroughly. Bring to boil. Cook for a minute.

5. Remove mixture from heat. Season with kosher salt and ground pepper. Add and stir eggs and cheese and mix. Combine the mixture with the broccoli. Transfer to 13x9" baking dish.

6. Bake at 325F for 1/2 hour. Serve hot.

Nutrition Information

Per Serving: 441 calories; 33 g fat; 15 g carbohydrates; 23.3 g protein; 148 mg cholesterol; 285 mg sodium

10 – Pepper Steak with Mushrooms

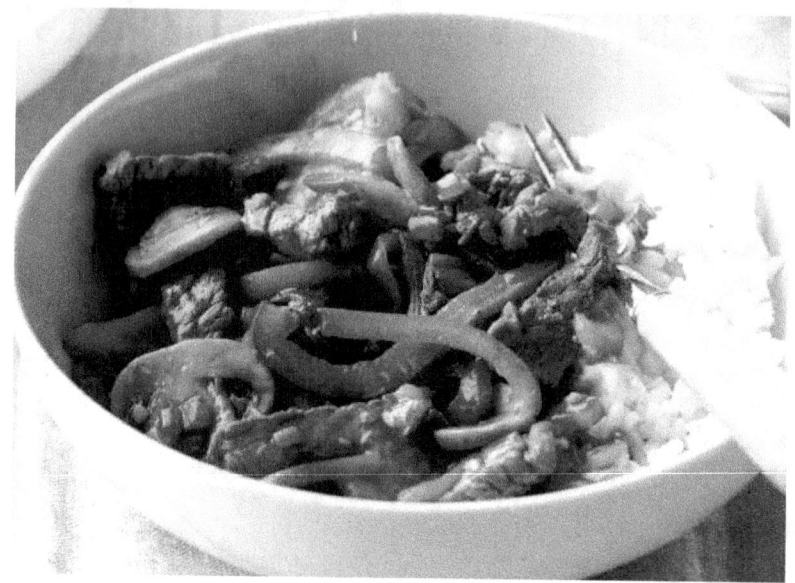

Ginger root, bell peppers and mushrooms offer lots of low-carb flavors in this stir fry. It's not as saucy as some tend to be, and it tastes great with hot rice.

Makes 4 Servings

Cooking + Prep Time: 45 minutes + 1 hour marinating time

Ingredients:

- 6 tbsp. of soy sauce, reduced sodium
- 1/8 tsp. of pepper, ground

- 1 lb. of thin-strip cut sirloin steak
- 1 tbsp. of corn starch
- 1/2 cup of beef broth, reduced-sodium
- 1 minced clove of garlic
- 1/2 tsp. of minced ginger root, fresh
- 3 tsp. of oil, canola
- 1 cup of julienne-cut sweet pepper, red
- 1 cup of julienne-cut pepper, green
- 2 cups of sliced mushrooms, fresh
- 2 wedge-cut tomatoes, medium
- 6 sliced green onions
- Optional: cooked rice, hot

Instructions:

1. Combine 3 tbsp. of soy sauce and ground pepper in shallow bowl. Add the beef. Turn and coat.

2. Cover bowl. Refrigerate for 1/2 hour to an hour. Combine broth, remaining soy sauce and corn starch in small sized bowl till smooth and set bowl aside.

3. Drain the beef and discard the marinade. In large wok or skillet, stir-fry ginger and garlic in 2 tsp. of oil for a minute.

Add beef. Stir-fry for four to six more minutes, till meat is not pink anymore. Remove the beef. Keep it warm.

4. Stir-fry peppers in the remainder of oil for a minute. Add the mushrooms. Stir-fry them for two more minutes, till peppers become tender-crisp.

5. Stir the broth mixture. Add to veggie mixture. Bring to boil. Stir while cooking for two minutes, till it thickens. Return the beef to the pan. Add the onions and tomatoes. Cook for two more minutes, till heated fully through. Serve on rice, if you like.

Nutrition Information

1-1/4 cups beef mixture:

10g fat (3g saturated fat),

241 calories,

841mg sodium,

64mg cholesterol,

5g sugars,

13g carbohydrate

25g protein

3g fiber,

11 – Slow Cooker Onion Pot Roast

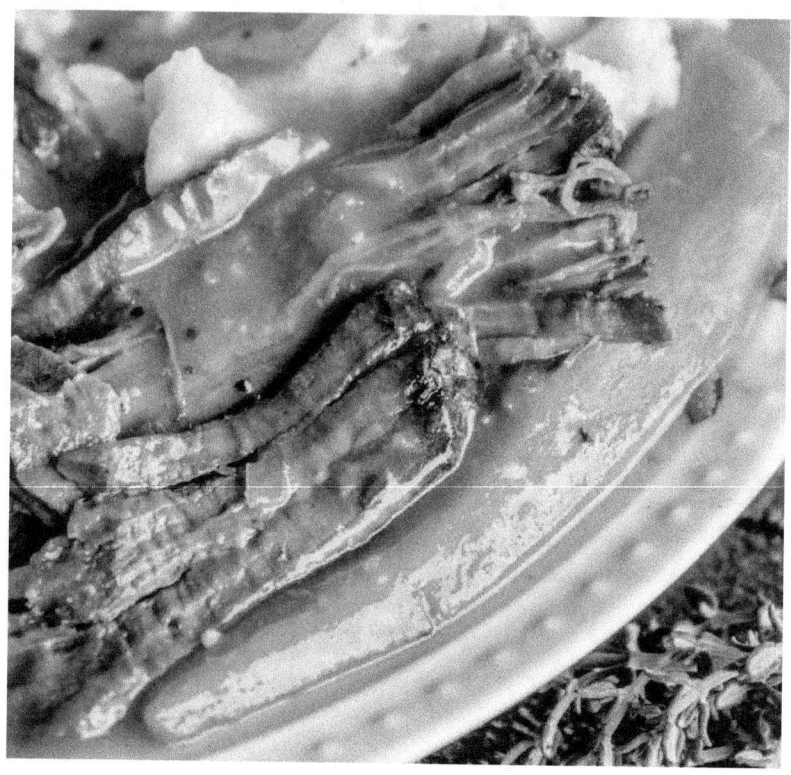

A delicious, healthy pot roast without a lot of work – it virtually **Makes** gravy on its own. If you don't have time to cook elaborate meals, toss the ingredients in a slow cooker and let it work for you.

Makes 12 Servings

Cooking + Prep Time: 10 minutes + 3-4 hours slow cooker time

Ingredients:

- 2 x 10 & 3/4-oz. cans of cream 'o mushroom soup, condensed
- 1 x 1-oz. pkg. of onion dry soup mix
- 1 & 1/8 cups of water, filtered
- 5 & 1/2 lbs. of pot roast

Instructions:

1. Mix water, soup and dry soup mix in slow cooker. Add pot roast. Coat with the soup. Cook on the HIGH setting for three to four hours. Serve.

Nutrition Information

Per Serving:

23.7 g fat;

426 calories;

45.6 g protein;

4.9 g carbohydrates;

639 mg sodium

127 mg cholesterol;

12 – Turkey Curry and Rice

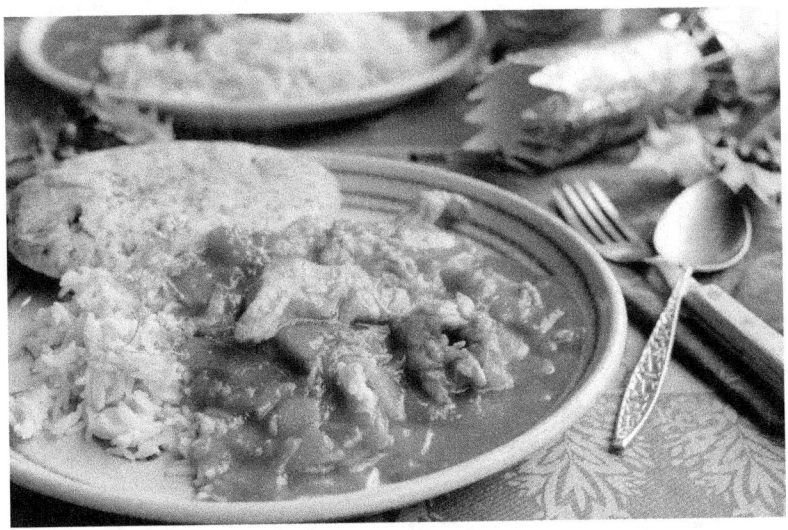

If you have some leftover turkey and you're hungry for a curry, this recipe brings them together in a tasty way. Turkey curry with cauliflower, carrots and special mango chutney over rice make a wonderful meal.

Makes 6 Servings

Cooking + Prep Time: 35 minutes

Ingredients:

- 1 & 1/3 cups of chicken broth, low sodium
- 2 tbsp. of curry powder

- 2 tbsp. of minced cilantro, fresh
- 3 minced cloves of garlic
- 3/4 tsp. of salt, kosher
- 1/2 tsp. of cardamom, ground
- 1/2 tsp. of ground pepper, black
- 3 sliced carrots, medium
- 1 chopped onion, medium
- 1 x 16-oz. pkg. of frozen, thawed cauliflower
- 3 cups of cooked turkey, chopped
- 1/2 cup of chutney, mango
- 2 tsp. of flour, all-purpose
- 1 cup of milk, coconut
- 4 & 1/2 cups of cooked rice, hot
- Optional: extra mango chutney, if desired

Instructions:

1. Mix first seven ingredients in large sized sauce pan. Add onion and carrots. Bring to boil.

2. Lower the heat. Cover and simmer for three to five minutes, till carrots are crisp but tender. Add the cauliflower. Cover and cook for four to six more minutes, till veggies become tender.

3. Stir in turkey and chutney and heat fully through. Mix coconut milk and flour in small sized bowl till mixture is smooth. Then stir this into the turkey mixture.

4. Stir constantly while bringing to boil. Stir and cook for one or two minutes, till the mixture thickens slightly. Serve with cooked rice. Add extra chutney, if desired.

Nutrition Information

1 cup turkey mixture with 3/4 cup rice:

9g fat (7g saturated fat),

363 calories,

787mg sodium,

1mg cholesterol,

16g sugars,

64g carbohydrate

7g protein,

5g fiber

13 – Grilled Asparagus

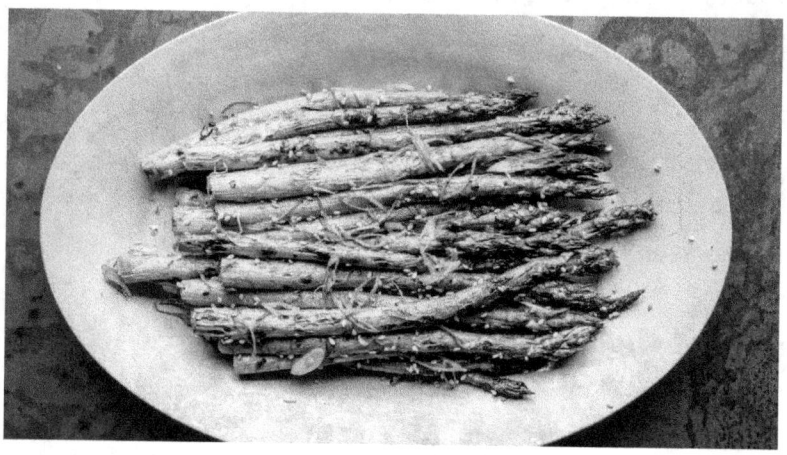

Grilled asparagus is a great dish to serve with baked fish or chicken. It's so tasty, and it's a healthy side dish.

Makes 4 Servings

Cooking + Prep Time: 45 minutes

Ingredients:

- 1 lb. of trimmed broccoli rabe
- 5 tbsp. of oil, olive
- 1 minced garlic clove
- 1 tbsp. of Parmesan cheese, grated

Instructions:

1. Bring large sized pot of lightly salted water to boil. Cut "X" in bottom of broccoli stems. Place in boiling water. Cook for about five minutes, till tender yet firm. Drain.

2. Heat oil in large skillet on med. heat. Sauté the garlic for one to two minutes. Add and stir broccoli rabe. Sauté for 10-15 minutes, until done as you desire. Dust using parmesan cheese, as desired. Serve.

Nutrition Information

Per Serving:

17.2 g fat;

192 calories;

4.5 g protein;

5.6 g carbohydrates;

53 mg sodium

1 mg cholesterol;

14 – Stuffed Zucchini

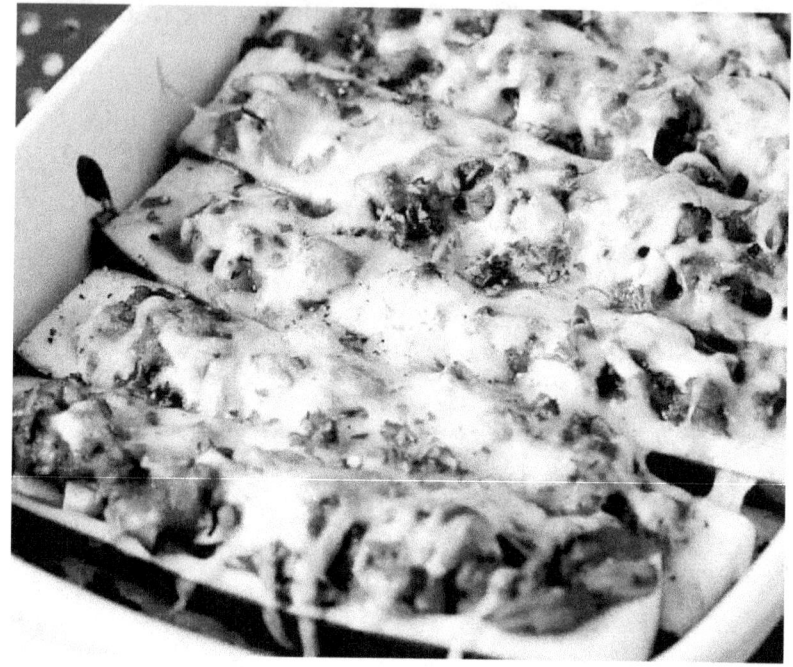

Sometimes I need to get creative to get the family to eat their vegetables. This stuffed zucchini uses pizza flavors that I KNOW they love, and it's healthy and low in calories, too.

Makes 6 Servings

Cooking + Prep Time: 1 hour

Ingredients:

- 6 x 8-oz. zucchini, medium
- 1 lb. of sausage links, Italian turkey, with removed casings
- 2 de-seeded, chopped tomatoes, medium
- 1 cup of bread crumbs, Japanese (panko)
- 1/3 cup of Parmesan cheese, grated
- 1/3 cup of minced parsley, fresh
- 2 tbsp. of minced oregano, fresh
- 2 tbsp. of minced basil, fresh
- 1/4 tsp. of pepper, ground
- 3/4 cup of mozzarella cheese shreds, part-skim
- Optional: extra minced parsley

Instructions:

1. Preheat the oven to 350F. Cut zucchinis in halves, lengthways. Scoop the pulp out and leave a 1/4" shell. Chop the pulp.

2. Place the zucchini shells in large sized microwavable dish. Cover and microwave in batches on the high setting for two to three minutes, till they are crisp but tender.

3. Cook zucchini pulp and sausage in large sized skillet on med. heat, for six to eight minutes, till sausage isn't pink anymore. Break the sausage into crumbles and drain.

4. Add and stir tomatoes, ground pepper, herbs, parmesan cheese and bread crumbs. Spoon the mixture into the zucchini shells.

5. Place shells in two 9x13-inch (ungreased) casserole dishes. Cover. Bake for 15-18 minutes or till the zucchini becomes tender. Then sprinkle with the mozzarella cheese.

6. Leave uncovered. Bake for five to eight minutes more, till cheese has melted. You can sprinkle with a bit more parsley, if you like. Serve.

Nutrition Information

2 stuffed zucchini halves:

9g fat (3g saturated fat),

206 calories,

485mg sodium,

39mg cholesterol,

5g sugars,

16g carbohydrate

17g protein

3g fiber,

15 – Garlic Chicken

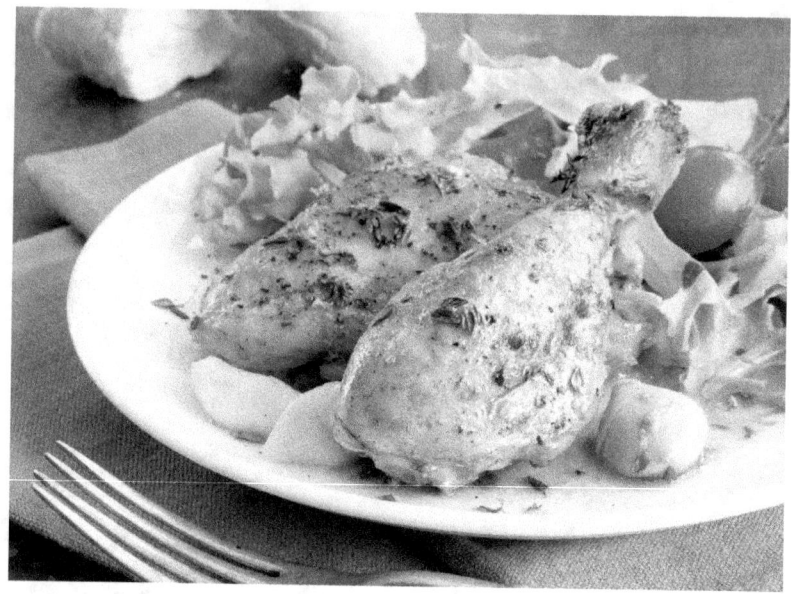

These two tastes just go together so well. It's easy to make and each bite offers garlic and breaded chicken. Everyone here loves it, and it's a healthy, low carb meal.

Makes 4 Servings

Cooking + Prep Time: 1 hour

Ingredients:

- 1/4 cup of oil, olive
- 2 crushed garlic cloves

- 1/4 cup of bread crumbs, Italian seasoned
- 1/4 cup of Parmesan cheese, grated
- 4 chicken breast halves, boneless, skinless

Instructions:

1. Preheat the oven to 425F.

2. Heat oil and crushed garlic in small sized sauce pan on low heat till warm. This typically takes a minute or two. Transfer oil and garlic to shallow bowl.

3. Combine Parmesan cheese and bread crumbs in another shallow bowl.

4. Dip the chicken breasts in olive oil and garlic mixture with tongs. Then transfer them to the breadcrumbs. Turn and coat evenly. Transfer the coated chicken to a baking dish.

5. Bake at 425F till juices are running clear and the meat isn't pink anymore. This usually takes a half-hour to 35 minutes. Internal temperature should be 165F or higher. Remove from oven and serve.

Nutrition Information

Per Serving:

16.8 g fat;

300 calories;

30.3 g protein;

5.7 g carbohydrates;

261 mg sodium

73 mg cholesterol;

16 – Pork Tacos

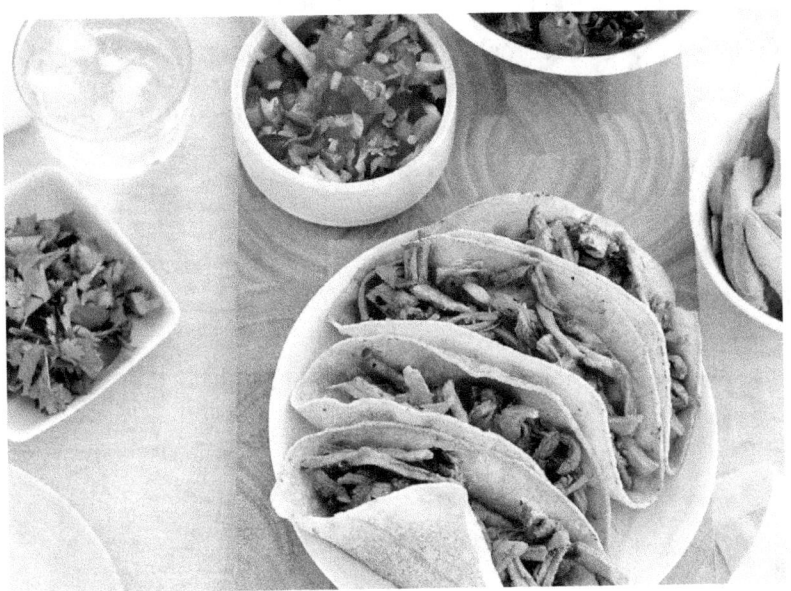

Need a new and tasty recipe for taco Tuesdays? Switch up the traditional beef, lettuce and cheese tacos for this healthier pork, apple and cilantro version. They're easy to make and taste great!

Makes 8 Servings

Cooking + Prep Time: 2 & 1/2 hours

Ingredients:

- 2 x 1-lb. pork tenderloins

- 1 x 12-oz. can of root beer

- For the slaw

- 12 oz. of red cabbage, shredded

- 2 julienned Granny Smith apples, medium

- 1/3 cup of vinegar, cider

- 1/4 cup of minced cilantro, fresh

- 1/4 cup of lime juice, fresh

- 2 tbsp. of sugar, granulated

- 1/2 tsp. of salt, kosher

- 1/2 tsp. of pepper, ground

For the assembly

- 1 x 18-oz. bottle of BBQ sauce

- 16 taco shells

Instructions:

1. Place the pork in medium sized slow cooker. Pour the root beer on top. Cover. Cook on low setting just till the meat is tender. Internal temperature should be 145F or higher. This usually takes between 2 & 2-1/2 hours.

2. In large sized bowl, toss the slaw ingredients. Cover and refrigerate till you're ready to serve.

3. Remove the tenderloins to a clean work space. Cover and let them sit for five minutes. Discard the cooking juices.

4. Chop the pork coarsely and return it to the slow cooker. Add and stir BBQ sauce and heat through. Fill taco shells with meat and top with slaw. Serve.

Nutrition Information

2 tacos with 1 cup slaw:

9g fat (2g saturated fat),

396 calories,

954mg sodium,

64mg cholesterol,

31g sugars,

53g carbohydrate

25g protein

3g fiber,

17 – Spinach and Mushrooms

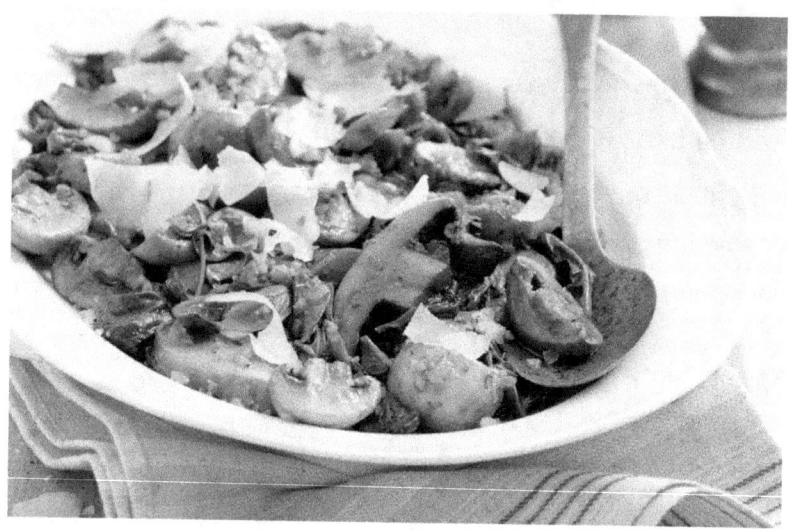

The inspiration for this dish comes from the Southern part of Italy. The mushrooms and spinach are sautéed with white wine, balsamic vinegar, garlic and onion. It's a low-calorie treat.

Makes 4 Servings

Cooking + Prep Time: 35 minutes

Ingredients:

- 4 tbsp. of oil, olive
- 1 chopped onion, small

- 2 chopped garlic cloves
- 14 oz. of sliced mushrooms, fresh
- 10 oz. of chopped spinach, fresh, cleaned
- 2 tbsp. of vinegar, balsamic
- 1/2 cup of wine, white
- Salt, kosher, as desired
- Black pepper, ground, as desired
- To garnish: chopped parsley, fresh

Instructions:

1. Heat oil in large sized skillet on med-high. Sauté garlic and onion in oil till they have started becoming tender.

2. Add mushrooms. Fry till they start shrinking. Toss in spinach. Stir constantly while frying for several minutes, till spinach wilts.

3. Stir constantly while adding vinegar till mixture absorbs it. Stir in wine. Reduce heat down to low. Simmer till mixture almost absorbs wine. Season as desired. Sprinkle with parsley and serve hot.

Nutrition Information

Per Serving:

14.2 g fat;

199 calories;

5.6 g protein;

10.3 g carbohydrates;

69 mg sodium

0 mg cholesterol;

18 – Basil and Lemon Salmon

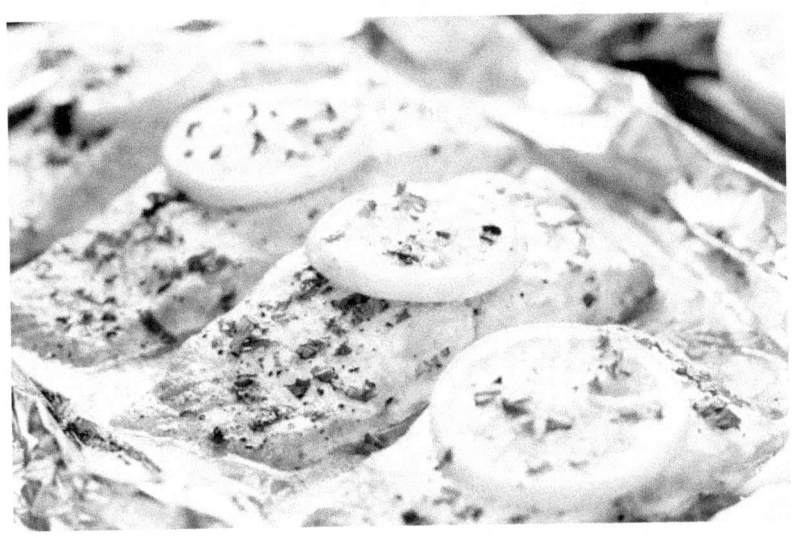

Salmon is a superfood, especially if you're on a diet. This salmon cooks easily in foil packets, which allows the tastes of the spices and herbs to shine through.

Makes 2 Servings

Cooking + Prep Time: 25 minutes

Ingredients:

- 2 x 5-oz. salmon fillets
- 1 tbsp. of melted butter, unsalted
- 1 tbsp. of minced basil, fresh

- 1 tbsp. of lemon juice, fresh
- 1/8 tsp. of salt, kosher
- 1/8 tsp. of pepper, ground
- Optional: lemon wedges, fresh

Instructions:

1. Prepare the grill for med. heat. Place fillets with skin side facing down on foil square.

2. Mix the lemon juice, basil, melted butter, kosher salt and ground pepper and spoon it over the salmon. Fold the foil around the fish and tightly seal it.

3. Cook on covered grill till fish can be flaked easily with fork. This generally takes 12 to 15 minutes. Then open the foil square carefully so steam can escape. Serve with the lemon wedges, if desired.

Nutrition Information

1 fillet:

19g fat

274 calories,

86mg cholesterol,

6g saturated fat,

1g carbohydrate

264mg sodium,

0 fiber,

0 sugars,

24g protein

19 – Chicken Zoodle Soup

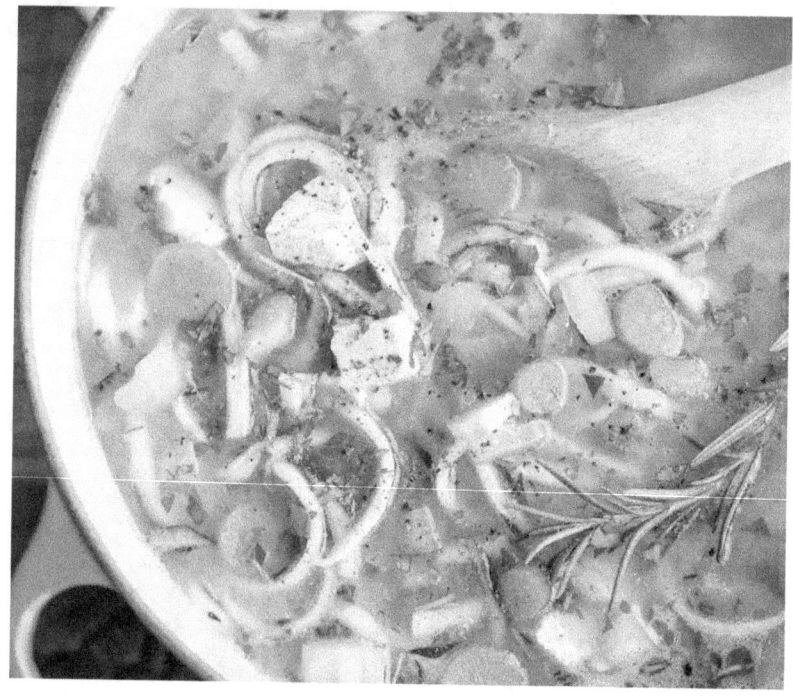

When the weather turns colder, my family loves soup. This recipe is healthier than chicken noodle soup, since zoodles are made from grated or spiralized zucchini. It has a texture like pasta, but not the carbs.

Makes 6 Servings

Cooking + Prep Time: 50 minutes

Ingredients:

- 2 tbsp. of oil, olive
- 1 cup of onions, diced
- 1 cup of celery, diced
- 3 cloves of minced garlic
- 5 x 14 & 1/2 oz. cans of chicken broth, low sodium
- 1 cup of carrots, sliced
- 3/4 lb. of bite-size cubed chicken breast, cooked
- 1/2 tsp. of basil, dried
- 1/2 tsp. of oregano, dried
- Optional: 1 pinch of thyme, dried
- Salt, kosher, as desired
- Pepper, ground, as desired
- 3 spiralized zucchini squash – you can use a veggie peeler if you don't have a spiralizer

Instructions:

1. Heat the oil in large sized pot on med-high. Sauté the garlic, onion and celery in the hot oil till barely tender, about three to five minutes.

2. Pour the chicken broth in pot. Add the chicken, carrots, kosher salt, ground pepper, thyme, oregano and basil.

3. Bring broth to boil. Reduce the heat down to med-low. Simmer the mixture till veggies become tender, about 18-22 minutes.

4. Divide the zucchini noodles (aka zoodles) in six individual bowls. Ladle broth over zoodles. Serve.

Nutrition Information

Per Serving:

9.5 g fat;

208 calories;

21.6 g protein;

8.9 g carbohydrates;

257 mg sodium

48 mg cholesterol;

20 – Ham and Asparagus Dinner

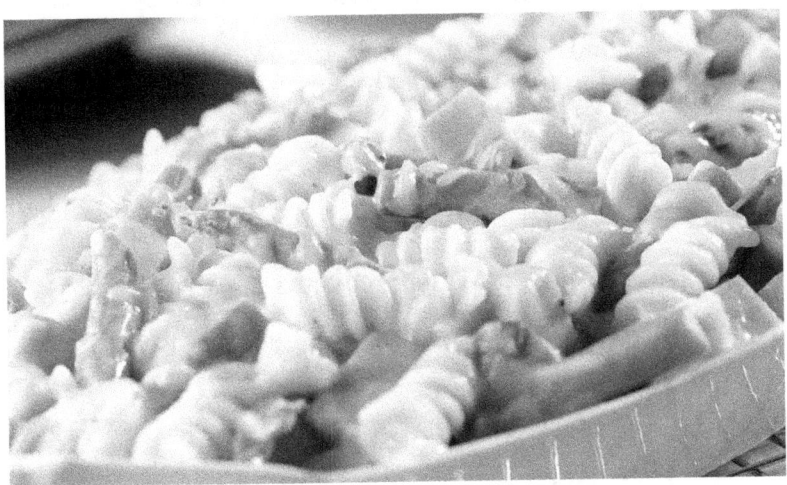

This ham dinner is a low fat favorite in my home. I've made it for years. With its ham chunks, tomato and asparagus, the tastes blend together well.

Makes 6 Servings

Cooking + Prep Time: 1/2 hour

Ingredients:

- 2 cups of spiral or corkscrew pasta, uncooked
- 3/4 lb. of 1-inch cubed asparagus, fresh
- 1 julienne-cut sweet pepper, yellow, medium
- 1 tbsp. of oil, olive

- 6 diced tomatoes, medium
- 6 oz. of cubed ham, fully cooked, boneless
- 1/4 cup of minced parsley, fresh
- 1/2 tsp. of salt, kosher
- 1/2 tsp. of oregano, dried
- 1/2 tsp. of basil, dried
- 1/8 – 1/4 tsp. of pepper, cayenne
- 1/4 cup of Parmesan cheese shreds

Instructions:

1. Cook the pasta using instructions on the package.

2. Sauté yellow sweet pepper and asparagus in large skillet till crisp but tender. Add the ham and tomatoes and heat them through.

3. Drain the pasta and add it to veggie mixture. Add and stir seasonings and parsley. Sprinkle with the Parmesan cheese. Serve.

Nutrition Information

1-1/3 cups:

5g fat (1g saturated fat),

204 calories,

561mg sodium,

17mg cholesterol,

5g sugars,

29g carbohydrate

12g protein

3g fiber,

21 – Radicchio Salmon Wraps

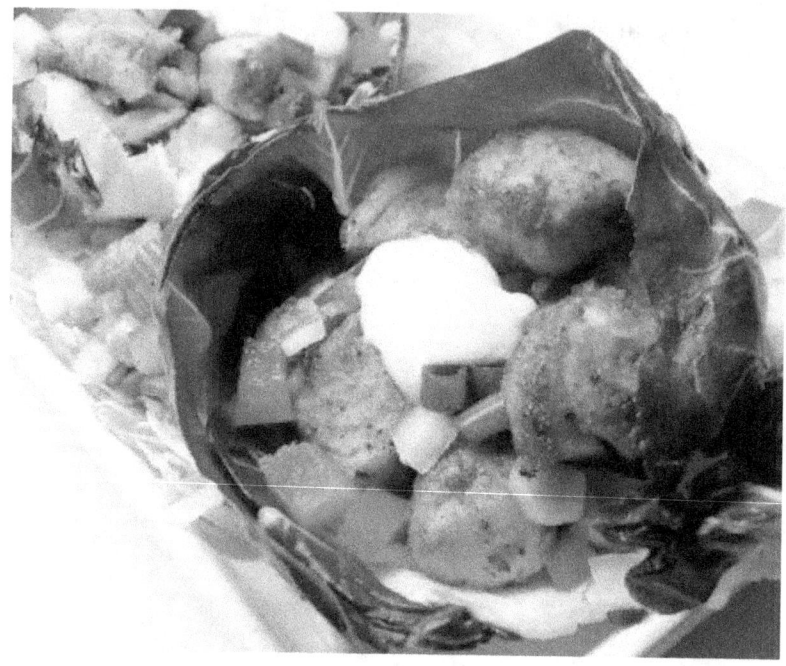

The Greek yogurt and salmon in this recipe offer heart-healthy Omega 3's. The bell peppers, radicchio and tomatoes have lycopene. This is a healthy meal that tastes great!

Makes 4 Servings

Cooking + Prep Time: 35 minutes

Ingredients:

For the Pico de Gallo

- 1 de-seeded, diced tomato
- 1/2 de-seeded, diced bell pepper, red
- 1/2 chopped onion, red
- 1 juiced lime, fresh

For the Cream Sauce

- 2/3 cup of plain yogurt, Greek
- 2 tbsp. of milk, skim
- 1/2 tsp. of seasoning blend
- For the Wraps
- 1 lb. of chunk-cut grilled salmon, skinless
- 12 radicchio leaves, whole

Instructions:

1. Combine the lime juice, onion, bell pepper and tomato in small sized bowl. Mix to create your Pico de Gallo sauce.

2. To prepare the cream sauce, whisk the skim milk, seasoning blend and yogurt together.

3. Place some chunks of grilled salmon in radicchio leaf. Top them with Pico de Gallo and then cream sauce. Repeat with the rest of the salmon and the radicchio leaves. Serve.

Nutrition Information

Per Serving:

17.6 g fat;

306 calories;

28.4 g protein;

7.5 g carbohydrates;

104 mg sodium

79 mg cholesterol;

22 – Egg Rolls and Noodles

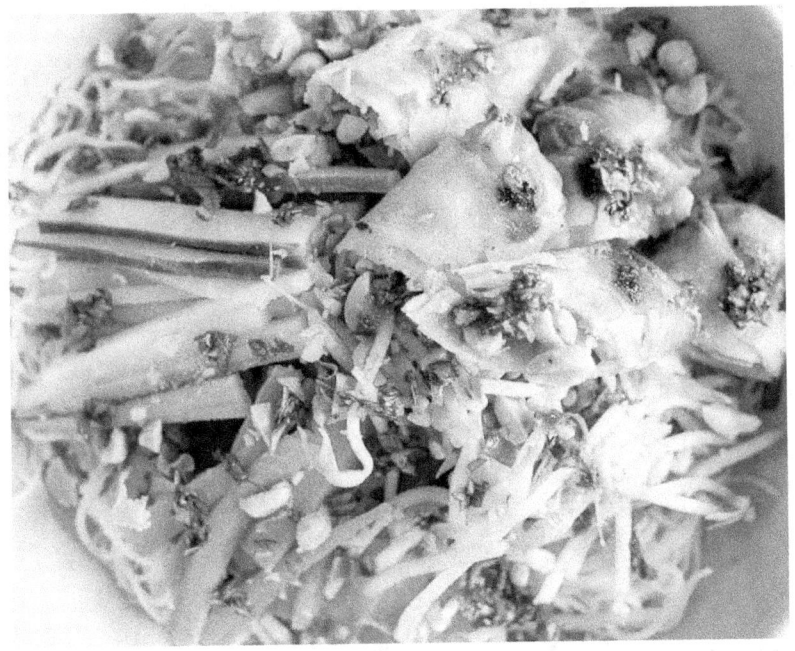

I love Asian style egg rolls, but they usually take a long time to make. So, I utilize this simpler recipe, which has deconstructed egg rolls in bowls on a stove top.

Makes 4 Servings

Cooking + Prep Time: 35 minutes

Ingredients:

- 1 tbsp. of oil, sesame

- 1/2 lb. of pork, ground
- 1 tbsp. of soy sauce, low sodium
- 1 minced clove of garlic
- 1 tsp. of ginger, ground
- 1/2 tsp. of salt, kosher
- 1/4 tsp. of turmeric, ground
- 1/4 tsp. of pepper, ground
- 6 cups of cabbage, shredded
- 2 shredded carrots, large
- 4 oz. of noodles, rice
- 3 thin-sliced green onions
- Optional: extra soy sauce, as desired

Instructions:

1. In heavy, large skillet, heat the oil on med-high. Cook while crumbling the pork till it browns, about four to six minutes.

2. Add and stir garlic, seasonings and soy sauce. Add the carrots and cabbage. Cook till the vegetables become tender, while occasionally stirring, for about four to six more minutes.

3. Cook the rice noodles using the directions on the package. Drain them and add immediately to the pork mixture. Toss and combine well.

4. Sprinkle with the green onions. Serve with extra soy sauce, as desired.

Nutrition Information

1-1/2 cups:

12g fat (4g saturated fat),

302 calories,

652mg sodium,

38mg cholesterol,

2g sugars,

33g carbohydrate

14g protein

4g fiber,

23 – Chicken Fajitas

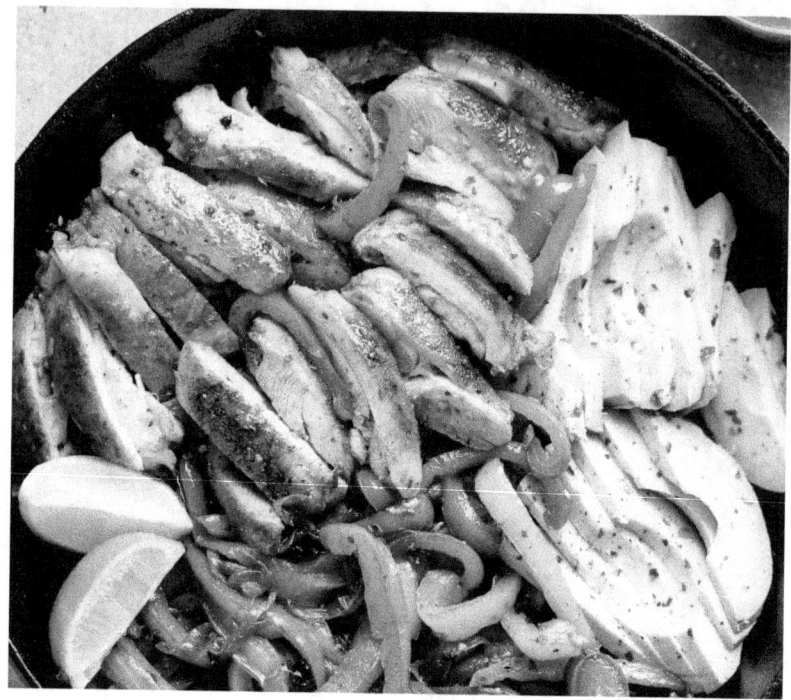

This is not your everyday chicken fajita. It's tangier! You can serve it with rice, beans, guacamole and all kinds of healthy add-ons, if you like.

Makes 6 Servings

Cooking + Prep Time: 35 minutes + 3-6 hours marinating time

Ingredients:

- 1/2 cup of oil, olive
- 1/2 cup of vinegar, white, distilled
- 1/2 cup of lime juice, fresh
- 2 small pkgs. of salad dressing mix, Italian flavor, dry
- 3 cubed chicken breasts, whole, skinless, boneless
- 1 sliced onion
- 1 sliced bell pepper, green

Instructions:

1. Combine lime juice, dressing mix, vinegar and oil in large sized glass bowl. Mix well.

2. Add the bell pepper, chicken strips and onion. Cover the dish. Place in the fridge for three to six hours to marinate.

3. Heat oil in large sized skillet. Remove the bell pepper, chicken and onion from the marinade. Sauté them in oil till onion becomes translucent and chicken has cooked completely through. Serve.

Nutrition Information

Per Serving:

18.8 g fat;

257 calories;

14.1 g protein;

7.7 g carbohydrates;

1101 mg sodium.

34 mg cholesterol;

24 – Pork Chops with Mushrooms

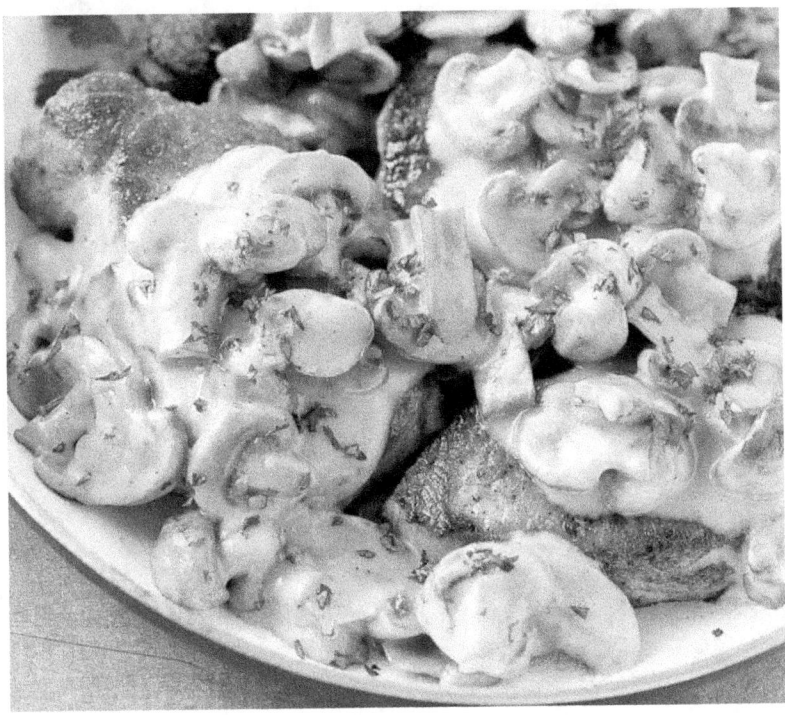

This recipe starts with boneless pork chops that are topped with a wonderful mushroom sauce. It's quick to make, but SO good! We serve it over brown rice.

Makes 4 Servings

Cooking + Prep Time: 45 minutes

Ingredients:

- 4 pork chops
- Salt, kosher, as desired
- Pepper, ground, as desired
- 1 pinch of garlic salt +/- as desired
- 1 chopped onion
- 1/2 lb. of sliced mushrooms, fresh
- 1 x 10 & 3/4 oz. can of cream o' mushroom soup, condensed

Instructions:

1. Season the pork chops as desired with kosher salt, ground pepper and/or garlic salt.

2. Brown pork chops on med-high in large sized skillet. Add mushrooms and onion. Sauté for about a minute.

3. Pour soup over the pork chops. Cover skillet. Reduce heat to med-low. Simmer for 20-30 minutes, till chops cook through completely. Serve.

Nutrition Information

Per Serving:

8.5 g fat;

210 calories;

23.6 g protein;

9.6 g carbohydrates;

924 mg sodium

65 mg cholesterol;

25 – Healthy Pizza

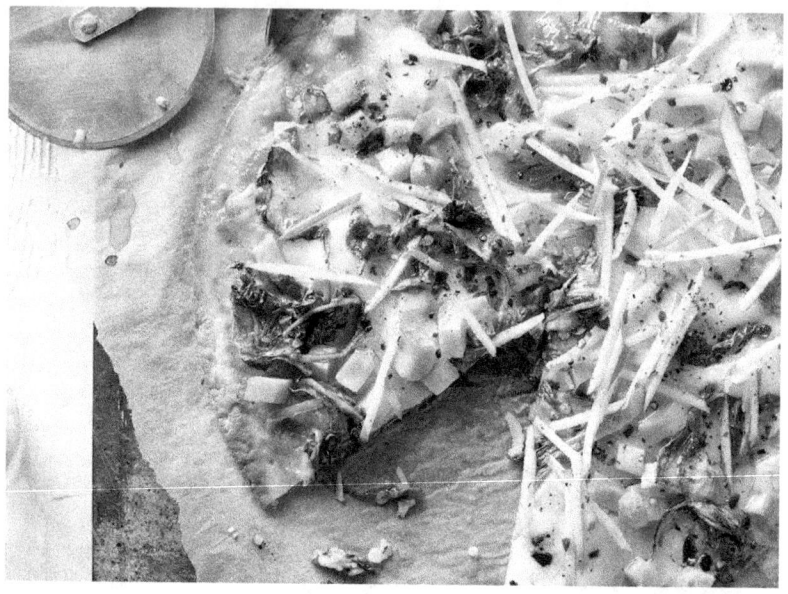

Wow, satisfying, mouth-watering AND healthy! It has all the pizza flavors everyone loves on a cheesy, crunchy, low carb crust. It's a win-win.

Makes 2-4 Servings

Cooking + Prep Time: 35 minutes

Ingredients:

For the crust

- 5 & 1/2 ounces of shredded mozzarella cheese
- 3/4 cup of flour, almond
- 2 tbsp. of cream cheese
- 1 tsp. of vinegar, white wine
- 1 egg, large
- 1/2 tsp. of salt, kosher
- Oil, olive, for greasing

For the Toppings

- 8 ounces of Italian sausage, fresh
- 1 tbsp. of butter, unsalted
- 1/2 cup of tomato sauce, unsweetened
- 1/2 tsp. of oregano, dried
- 3 & 1/2 ounces of shredded mozzarella cheese

Instructions:

1. Preheat oven to 400F.

2. Heat cream and mozzarella cheese in non-stick pan over med. heat. Stir till they have melted together. Add other ingredients. Combine well.

3. Grease your hands using olive oil. Flatten dough on baking paper. Make an 8-inch circle.

4. Prick crust all over with fork. Bake at 400F for about 10 to 12 minutes, till the coloring is a golden-brown, then remove crust from oven.

5. Sauté ground sausage in butter or olive oil.

6. Spread thin tomato sauce layer on pizza crust. Top with meat and cheese.

7. Bake for 12-15 minutes, till cheese is fully melted. Sprinkle with oregano. Serve.

Nutrition Information

Amount Per Serving

Total Fat: 20.5 g

Calories: 265.8

Sodium: 642.0 mg

Cholesterol: 42.7 mg

Dietary Fiber: 1.3 g

Total Carbs: 5.0 g

Protein: 17.6 g

Desserts on a diet? Sure, try these out...

26 – Carrot Cake

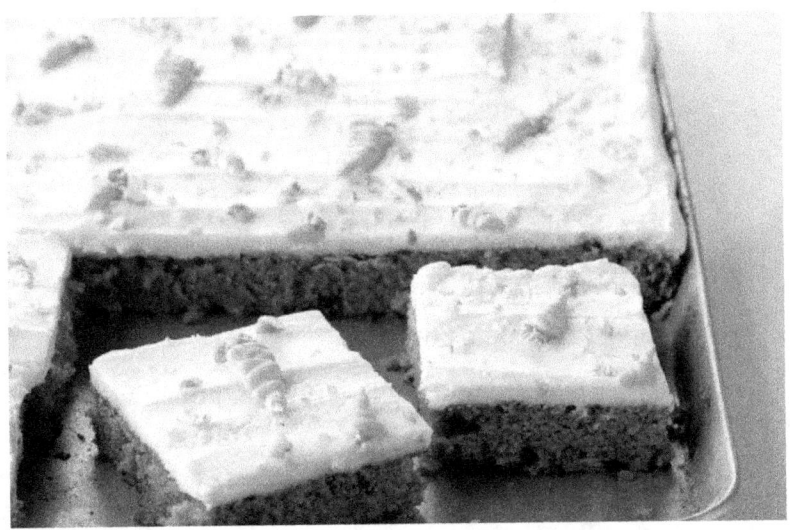

This is a lower fat version of the always popular carrot cake. It uses apple sauce, along with the carrots, and you top it off with pineapple, walnuts and raisins.

Makes 18 Servings

Cooking + Prep Time: 1 hour & 10 minutes

Ingredients:

- 6 eggs, large, whites only
- 1 & 1/3 cups of sugar, granulated
- 1 cup of apple sauce

- 1/2 cup of milk, skim
- 1 & 1/2 tsp. of vanilla extract, pure
- 1/4 tsp. of cloves, ground
- 1/2 tsp. of nutmeg, ground
- 1 tbsp. of cinnamon, ground
- 2 tsp. of baking soda
- 1 cup of flour, whole wheat
- 1 cup of flour, all-purpose
- 1 x 8-oz. can of pineapple, crushed, juice included
- 2 cups of carrots, shredded
- 1/2 cup of walnuts, chopped
- 1/2 cup of raisins

Instructions:

1. Preheat the oven to 350F. Grease 13x9" pan lightly with non-stick spray.

2. Beat egg whites in large sized bowl. Beat in sugar slowly, then beat in vanilla, apple sauce and skim milk.

3. Add and stir flours, baking soda, cinnamon, nutmeg and cloves.

4. Stir in, one after another, pineapple and juice, raisins, carrots and walnuts. Pour into pan prepared in step 1.

5. Bake for 35 to 40 minutes at 350F. Toothpick in middle will come back clean when it is done. Serve.

Nutrition Facts

Per Serving:

2.4 g fat;

167 calories;

3.9 g protein;

34.1 g carbohydrates;

171 mg sodium

< 1 mg cholesterol;

27 – Crunchy Chocolate Bars

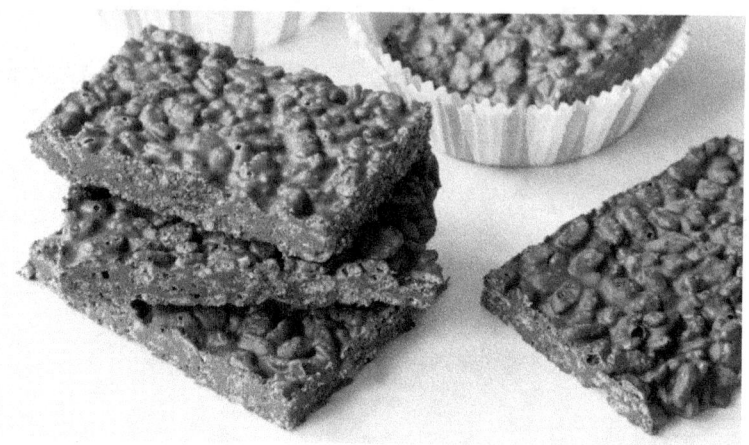

It's not easy to find reduced calorie chocolate chips, so stock up when you find them. They are an integral part of this chocoholic's dream. You can use regular chocolate chips if you have to but use less.

Makes 24 Servings

Cooking + Prep Time: 15 minutes

Ingredients:

- 6 cups of crispy rice cereal, chocolate flavor
- 1 & 1/2 tbsp. of margarine
- 1 & 1/2 tbsp. of peanut butter, reduced fat
- 8 oz. of marshmallows, large

- 1/3 cup of semi-sweet chocolate morsels, reduced fat

Instructions:

1. Spray 13x9" baking dish with a non-stick type spray.

2. Place rice cereal in large sized bowl.

3. Combine margarine, peanut butter and marshmallows in sauce pan. Stir constantly while cooking on low till marshmallows melt completely.

4. Pour that mixture over cereal. Stir till coated well.

5. Add, then mix in the chocolate morsels.

6. Press mixture in pan prepared in step 1. Spread it out with a spatula. Slice in 24 bars. Serve.

Nutrition Information

Amount Per Serving

Total Fat: 4.1 g

Calories: 99.4

Sodium: 41.6 mg

Cholesterol: 7.6 mg

Dietary Fiber: 0.4 g

Total Carbs: 16.8 g

Protein: 0.9 g

28 – Spiced Apples

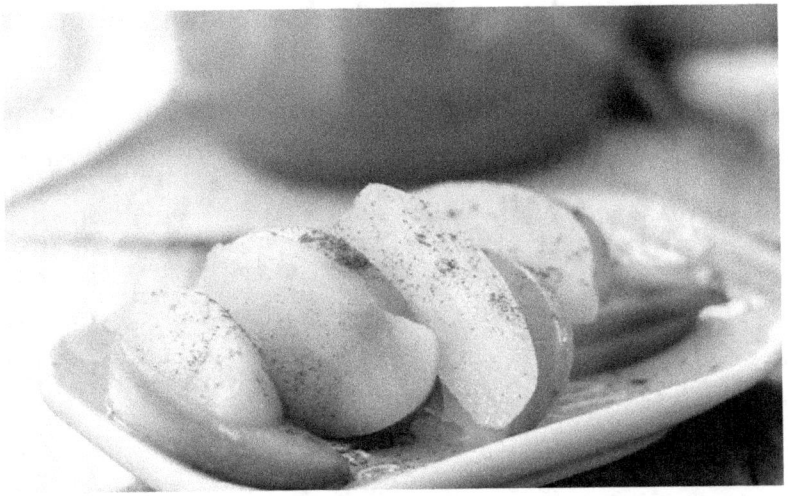

These apples dress up any holiday tabletop! The spices in the candy work wonders for the apples. You can decrease or increase the spice and color by adding less or more candy.

Makes 8 Servings

Cooking + Prep Time: 25 minutes

Ingredients:

- 8 apples, Granny Smith
- 2 tbsp. of Splenda®
- 1 tsp. of lemon juice, fresh
- 1/4 cup of red hot cinnamon candy

Instructions:

1. Peel the apples, then remove the cores and slice them.

2. Place all the ingredients in a microwave-safe medium bowl. Microwave on the high setting for 12-15 minutes. Stir every five minutes.

3. Cover bowl with cling wrap. Allow to cool - or you can serve them warm.

Nutrition Facts

Per Serving:

0.2 g fat;

110 calories;

0.4 g protein;

28.8 g carbohydrates;

4 mg sodium

0 mg cholesterol;

29 – Berry Crisp

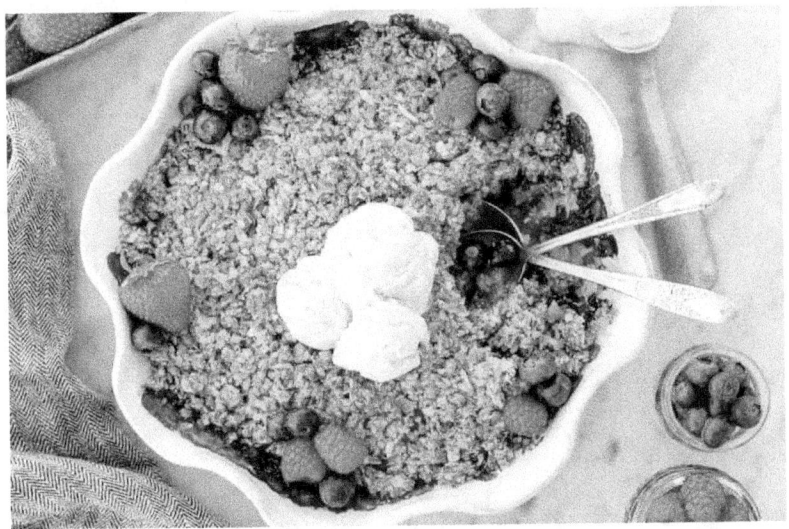

The fruit filling in this recipe is SO tasty. You can make it with fewer spices, if you like. The topping is as crusty as it is crumb-like, but it **Makes** a wonderful texture.

Makes 6 Servings

Cooking + Prep Time: 50 minutes

Ingredients:

For the fruit

- 1 x 16-oz. bag mixed berries, frozen

- 1 x 7/8-oz. box of Jell-O® vanilla pudding mix, sugar free, cook & serve type
- 1 tsp. of cinnamon, ground
- 1/2 tsp. of nutmeg, ground
- 1/4 cup of milk, nonfat

For the crisp

- 1 & 1/2 cups of oats, old fashioned
- 1/2 cup of Splenda®
- 8 oz. of plain yogurt, fat-free
- 1 tsp. of almond extract, pure

Instructions

1. Spray 8" square baking pan with non-stick spray.

2. Mix fruits in pan. Stir thoroughly.

3. Mix crisp ingredients in separate bowl.

4. Spread crisp mixture over berries.

5. Bake in 350F oven for 40 to 45 minutes. Topping should be crunchy. Serve.

Nutrition Information

Amount Per Serving

Total Fat 4.2 g

Calories 216.2

Polyunsaturated Fat 0.9 g

Saturated Fat 1.6 g

Cholesterol 5.1 mg

Monounsaturated Fat 1.1 g

Potassium 162.7 mg

Sodium 15.5 mg

Dietary Fiber 6.1 g

Total Carbohydrate 40.1 g

Protein 6.2 g

Sugars 4.9 g

30 – Pear with Cinnamon Frozen Yogurt

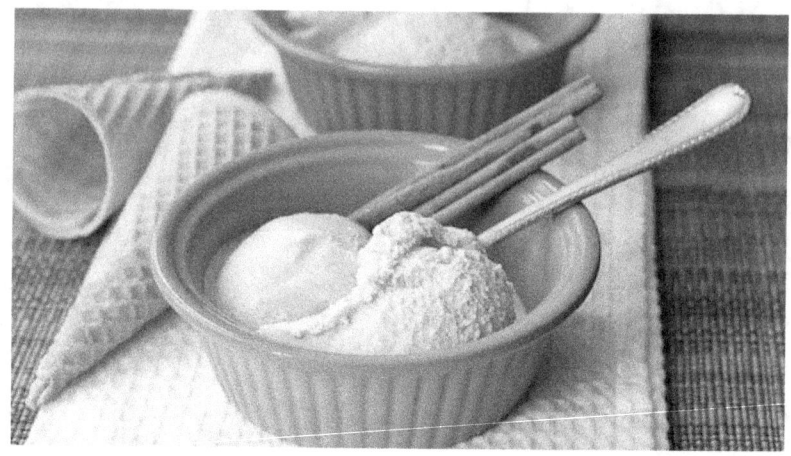

This dessert has no added sugar, and still luscious. The spiced apple cider flavor is accented with the taste of ginger bread. We love it regardless of the season.

Makes 8 Servings

Cooking + Prep Time: 50 minutes

Ingredients:

- 1 x 15-oz. can of halved pears
- 2 cups of yogurt, vanilla
- 1/3 cup of Splenda®

- 1/2 tsp. of cinnamon, ground
- 1/4 tsp. of allspice, ground

Instructions:

1. Drain the pears. Reserve 1/2 cup juice. Puree the pears in a food processor.

2. Combine the pears, yogurt, reserved pear juice, sugar, allspice and cinnamon in the canister of an ice cream maker. Freeze using the instructions of manufacturer. Serve when frozen.

Nutrition Information

Per Serving:

0.8 g fat;

111 calories;

3.2 g protein;

23.7 g carbohydrates;

43 mg sodium

3 mg cholesterol;

Conclusion

This diet-conscious cookbook has shown you…

… How to use healthy, low calorie and/or low carb ingredients to affect unique tastes in dishes both well-known and rare.

How can you include diet recipes in your home repertoire?

You can…

- Make sweet but not sugary breakfasts and savory breakfasts, too, without adding calories or carbs. These are just as tasty as the full-sugar equivalents.
- Learn to cook with healthy fruits – preferably the ones that are low in natural sugars – to make great tasting treats for your family.
- Enjoy making the delectable seafood and meat dishes you love. Fish is a mainstay in the realm of diet meals, and there are SO many ways to make it great.
- Make dishes using healthy vegetables, which are often used in cooking diet meals.

- Make various types of sugar-free or low sugar pastries like carrot cake and fruit sherbets that will tempt your family's sweet tooth.

Have fun experimenting! Enjoy the results!

www.ingramcontent.com/pod-product-compliance
Lightning Source LLC
Chambersburg PA
CBHW062046280526
45788CB00003B/1131